CW00926880

Essential Oils:

A-Z Essential Oils Reference for Health and Healing

Table of content

Introduction 3

Chapter 1 – Getting Started 5

The Wonder Oils 5

Peppermint 7

Lavender 8

Tea tree 10

Chapter 2 – The Best of the Blends 12

Chapter 3 – Oils by Symptoms or Desired Effect 17

Body Aches and Pains 18

Natural Cold and Flu Remedies..20

Stress..22

The Air of the House is the Mood of the Home 23

Chapter 4 – The Practical Side of Things 26

Essential Skin Care 27

For the Hair 29

Weight Loss and Weight Management 30

Chapter 5 – The Tricks of the Trade: How to Use Essential Oils....................................33

Diffusing 34

Taking the Oil Internally 36

Conclusion 38

FREE Bonus Reminder 40

Introduction

If you have spent any amount of time online, you know that it is important to watch what you are putting in or on your body. You know that there are medications and supplements that are meant to help your health in a variety of ways, but then you read that you should avoid a whole list of items that are then found in the supplements you are using.

So what do you do?

You know that you want to do the best thing for your health and your body, but what are you supposed to do when the very things you are supposed to use for your health end up being full of the very things you try to avoid.

You think of how you want to do what is best for your health, for your family, and for the planet, but you don't think you can do this if you are supporting the synthetic products that are on the shelves today.

This is a common feeling that a lot of people share, and thankfully the number one solution to this problem is also the solution to your health concerns. Essential oils are entirely natural, free of harmful synthetic chemicals, and can be used in more ways than any synthetic medication you could imagine.

You have a headache, you want to relax, and you want to settle the house down at the end of the day.

You don't want to turn to the synthetic medications that are full of warnings and things to watch for, but what do you do?

Essential oils is the answer. You can diffuse a few drops in a diffuser, you can apply a few drops directly to your skin, or you can even add certain kinds to tea, and you get the same great results.

Calm, quiet tranquility fills your home, and you feel better.

That's just the beginning. The more familiar you get with essential oils, the more you will be able to treat the ailments that arise, and the more natural you can live.

So are you ready to jump into the world of essential oils?

Naturally.

Chapter 1 – Getting Started

There is a lot of excitement when you start out in this journey, but before you just dive in and spread oils on everything, I want to get you started on the right track. This means you need to know what you are doing from the beginning.

You can't just toss essential oils around and see what happens, you have to know what each oil does, and how to use them for your particular symptoms. This is something you can use both ways. You can use this knowledge to use the right oil for your particular ailment, and you can avoid the oils that won't help you or potentially make you feel worse.

On the other hand, if you know what oils create different results, you will be able to set up your home with a lot of preventative aspects, meaning you won't get sick as often or feel the stress to begin with.

So, let's dive in and learn the facts about essential oils, how to use them, and what oils work well with each other.

Knowledge is an effective weapon.

The Wonder Oils

While each section you find is going to have its own list of oils, there are a few oils that seem to stand out from the rest. Yes, there are going to be times when you need to treat something specific, and you will need an equally specific oil to get the job done, but on the other hand, you are going to see a few oils show up time and time again, no matter what the ailment happens to be.

These are the oils I would like to refer to as the Wonder Oils, because there are so many ways using these oils can make your life better.

They are good for the specifics, and they are good for the broad categories.

Whether you are dealing with aches, pains, illness, insomnia, or want to promote things such as peace, tranquility, focus, happiness, and better relationships, these are the oils you always want to have on hand.

Peppermint

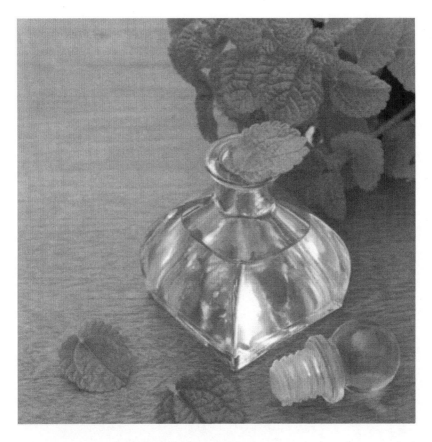

While many of us may associate this scent and taste with the holidays, there are a few things you need to know about this delightful oil that has nothing to do with Christmas trees or Santa Clause.

Peppermint oil has a light, fresh scent that blends exceptionally well with most other oils. It can be diffused for aroma therapy, applied topically on various aches and pains, and it can be enjoyed internally if it is highly diluted in water or tea. This oil is going to ease pains, clear your mind, and make you feel better and at peace.

It is abundantly available... you can purchase it not only online but in a variety of health and wellness stores to even large chain department stores. This oil truly is a wonder worker, and I suggest you keep plenty of it on hand at all times.

Lavender

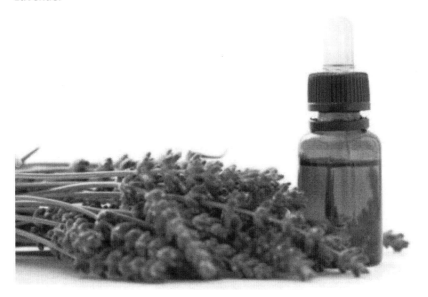

The floral scent of lavender is soothing to the mind, body, and soul. You would be amazed at how many people there are who think they don't like floral scents, but gravitate toward lavender.

Certainly among the best of the best, lavender is easily considered a Wonder Oil.

This oil is like peppermint in regards to the fact it will ease many of your life's ailments. Whether you are tense, stressed, or unable to sleep, a few drops of this oil spread across your forehead, blended into your bath water, or diffused in your bedroom is going to ease all of that tension that has built up and help you not only fall asleep, but stay asleep.

When you realize you can't become dependent on it, but you can use it as freely as you like, you are going to realize even more why you should keep this on hand at all times.

Make a space in your cabinet to house your lavender, peppermint, and tea tree oils, and there are few things you will face that you won't be able to handle.

Tea tree

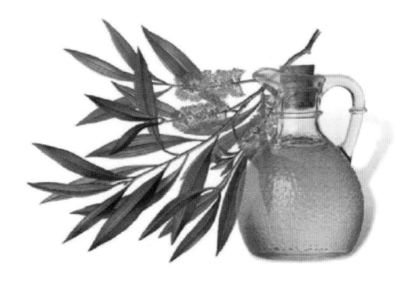

When it comes to physical ailments and imperfections, few things are going to do more for you than tea tree oil. While this oil has a strong, somewhat overwhelming scent, the benefits it does for your skin are far beyond the strong scent it holds.

Tea tree oil is a natural antiseptic. You can apply it to scrapes, cuts, and even acne and it will heal and clear up the imperfection. Excellent for hair, skin, and even sore throats and coughs, this oil is best diffused into the air for aroma therapy or mixed with a carrier oil and applied topically.

If you want to lighten the scent of this Wonder Oil, you can blend it with less offensive oils such as lavender, rose, or lemon. Another terrific benefit that comes with tea tree oil is that it is even more abundant than peppermint or lavender. You can purchase large vials of the purest form online or in health food stores, and it doesn't cost nearly as much as some of the more exotic oils do.

This oil's benefits far outweigh the scent, so make sure to get a large vial of it and keep it up in your cabinet along with the lavender and peppermint. You will be so glad you did.

Chapter 2 – The Best of the Blends

You may only be experiencing one feeling, or you may want to promote a singular feeling, in which case you only need to choose the oil or oils that you enjoy. There are going to be times, however, when you need to address more than one problem at a time, or when you want to create a blend of energy in your home.

To do this, you need to combine oils in properly to get the desired effect.

Thankfully, blending oils is not only easy, it is encouraged to create the best fragrances and optimum results, so you won't have any problem at all finding the right blend for your needs.

The trick to getting the best of the blends is to know how to blend the oils yourself

If you get online, you are going to find that there are plenty of blends all ready to go. The supplier puts them together and sells them as a blend, usually under the name of what you need it for.

For example, you can purchase an oil blend from Doterra called "On Guard". It is an immunity support oil, but if you look closer at it, you will see that it is, in fact, a blend of the everyday oils you have on hand such as wild orange, clove bud, cinnamon, eucalyptus, and rosemary.

While there is a lot of convenience to purchasing the oil already blended, you are going to find that you will save a lot of money, and get a lot more of the product if you purchase the oils separately and blend them yourself.

Wait, purchasing all of those oils separately isn't going to be inexpensive... the blend is a lot cheaper to buy as it is

Yes, that may be true, but if you think about it, if you purchase the ingredients separately, not only do you get enough to make the blend yourself, but you also get the extra oils left over to put to other use.

This is going to come in handy if you want to have the immunity support, as well as treat any ailment you already have, or simply to set some aside until you need it again. You see, when you are blending the oils yourself, you always have a lot of each on hand, simply because you only use a few drops of each one when you do use it.

So that brings us to the actual blending aspect.

When you blend the oils yourself, make sure you look at the total number of drops you are going to be using at the end result. If you are making enough to save some, keep the ratios the same, but if you are only mixing one time use at a time, watch out for how much you are actually using.

What this means is that if you are going to use the oils to make the equivalent to Doterra's On Guard, you need to realize that the 2 drops you use from that bottle are 2 blended drops.

I know that sounds confusing at first, but think about it this way. If you are mixing in the On Guard into your tea to sip on, you only need 1 or 2 drops to do it. All of those oils I listed that create this blend come together in those 2 drops you put into your tea.

If you were to take each of those drops and place only 1 drop each in your tea separately, then you will end up with 5 or 6 drops, which is simply too much to ingest at one time. If you put this all in your tea at once, you will run into problems from overdosing on the oils.

To get around this, you need to cut back on the amount of oils you are using in your tea, or (better yet) blend them all separately then take 2 drops of what you have blended. The most important thing you need to remember when it comes to essential oils is that you can overdose, and too much of some of them can be toxic.

Keep small jar glasses on hand, or purchase some of your own vials to store the extra oils you blend. This is going to keep them safe until you need them again, and help you stay on track with the proper dosage of the oils.

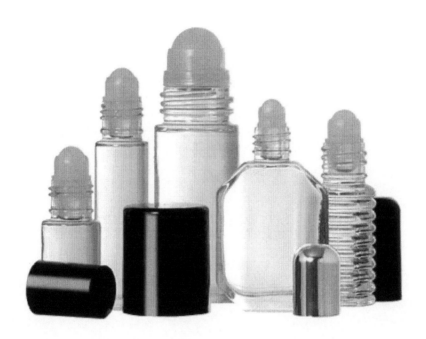

Small vials that have the drop lid are available online, or you can even get them locally at a number of stores. One of the major benefits to mixing your own blends in your own bottles is that you get to then choose the bottles you want to use as well.

This means you can create your own mists, roll ons, or drop bottles to suit your own taste, and keep them on hand where you want them. Say you want to take an anti-stress blend to work with you? No problem!

Purchase a roll on dispenser, mix up your favorite blend or just use your favorite anti-stress oil, fill your roll on dispense, and toss it in your purse. No matter where your day goes you will have your instant anti-stress mechanism at just an arm's length away, and your day is going to go so much better.

When you are creating your own blends, start with the desired effect you want your blend to have, and move on from there.

For example, if you want a blend that is going to help you sleep, but you also want to relieve tension and stress besides, start with the lavender. You want there to be more lavender in this blend than anything else, so I would recommend starting with 10 or 12 drops of this oil.

Then, pick the other oils you want. Peppermint is great for stress relief, so choose this one next, but don't put in the same amount. Perhaps 6 or 7 drops to suit your own taste.

What you want to keep in mind is that you want to use the most of your main focus, then add in the secondary oils as secondary benefits. Once you have this down, you can make any blend you want for any use you want.

Get creative!

Chapter 3 – Oils by Symptoms or Desired Effect

There are times when you are looking through the oils to see what they do, but there are also times when you feel a certain way and you want to find the oils that make it better.

What I mean by this is that you may enjoy the smell of rose oil and lavender oil, so you diffuse this in your home often. You are going to gain the amazing benefits that come from diffusing this oil... which means you are going to feel calm, relaxed, open, etc... but this doesn't help when you are suffering from a headache.

So, if you happen to have some sort of ailment (a headache, a stomach ache, a tooth ache), you need to know which oils to use specifically for these problems.

Here are oils separated into categories based on the symptoms you feel.

You can use one of the oils in the category, or you can mix and match as you please to take care of many of your symptoms.

Body Aches and Pains

Body aches and pains are annoying as well as debilitating. When you feel any of these symptoms, you know you want to get better as soon as possible.

I suggest for any of the oils or oil blends you use here, mix a few drops with a carrier oil and massage onto the aching area.

You can also add 10 to 12 drops into a warm bath and soak your pain away.

Headaches

Eucalyptus

Lavender

Peppermint

Stomach aches

Peppermint

Ginger

Roman chamomile

Melissa

Star anise

Grapefruit

Spearmint

Cardamom

Coriander

Fennel

Aniseed

Joint pain and stiffness

Sweet marjoram

Chamomile

Rosemary

Peppermint

Eucalyptus

Muscle cramps

Peppermint

Lemongrass

Basil

Vetiver

Sage

Cypress

Grapefruit

Rosemary

Natural Cold and Flu Remedies

When it comes to treating the cold and flu, I suggest you use a diffuser next to your bed or couch. The oils will fill the air and the aroma therapy will clear the illness right out.

If you are dealing with specific aches such as a sore throat, cough, or headache, you may also mix the oils of your choice with a carrier oil and massage it into the infected area, or add a drop or two to tea and sip on it.

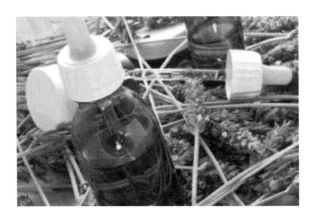

Colds

Lavender

Eucalyptus

Thyme

Rosemary

Garlic

Sandalwood

Lemon

Chamomile

Peppermint

Sore Throat

Eucalyptus

Oregano

Sage

Tea tree

Ginger

Peppermint

Cough

Lavender

Peppermint

Lemongrass

Frankincense

Lemon

Stress

No matter what kind of job you work or what kind of life you live, you are going to deal with a level of stress.

To rid your mind and body of that stress, I strongly suggest you use these oils or any blend of these oils in a diffuser, or add 10 to 12 drops into your hot bath water before you soak in the tub.

Tension

Helichrysum

Peppermint

Spearmint

Roman chamomile

Eucalyptus

Lavender

Insomnia

Lavender

Roman chamomile

Sweet marjoram

Vetiver

Ylang ylang

Anxiety

Basil

Clary sage

Bergamot

Frankincense

Ylang ylang

Marjoram

Peppermint

The Air of the House is the Mood of the Home

They say prevention is the best cure, and if you set up your home to be a safe haven, you are going to skip out on a lot of stressful symptoms that pop up in day to day life.

Use these oils in diffusers around your home. Diffusers aren't expensive and they are easy to maintain.

Prevent ailments and issues and promote peace and health with these oils blended into the air of your home at all times.

The Essentials you will need:

To promote tranquility

Chamomile

Roman chamomile

Lavender

Cedar wood

To promote happiness

Orange

Rose

Jasmine

Ginger

Cloves

Sandalwood

Petitgrain

Frankincense

Lemon

Geranium

To promote energy

Black pepper

Bergamot

Grapefruit

Peppermint

Rosemary

Thyme

Lemon

Basil

Fennel

To promote peace

Tangerine

Orange

Patchouli

Ylang ylang

Cassia

Davana

German chamomile

Cistus

Lavender

Lemon

Chapter 4 – The Practical Side of Things

In life there are far more things we want to address and take care of besides mood and colds. You want beautiful hair, you want to lose weight or maintain a weight loss. Your teenagers want clear skin and you want to avoid or get rid of the wrinkles that somehow appeared around your mouth and eyes.

Sure, it's great to know how to address a headache or sleeplessness, but once you know how to also get rid of such things as acne, wrinkles, and oily hair, you are going to be completely taken care of in your oil usage.

That is why I have included this chapter, so you know exactly what you can use to treat or prevent those physical imperfections you don't want to have to deal with any longer.

And when you combine the fact you get to save money as well as save your skin from harmful chemicals, you have a complete win, and everyone wants to have that.

Essential Skin Care

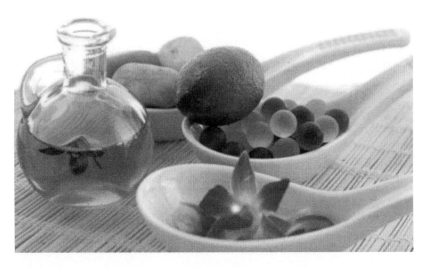

People of all ages across the globe spend hundreds and thousands of dollars each year on various skin care products. Each of the products claim they are going to do the magic trick, but most of them end up not working anyway.

Not to mention these products are full of chemicals you don't want on your skin. Using essential oils are always a better choice, and I promise you that you are going to see better results using these than you ever did with store products.

To use these, mix with your face soap, moisturizer, or with a carrier oil and apply directly to the spot you want to focus on.

How to get rid of acne

Jojoba

Lavender

Tea tree

Orange

Frankincense

Get rid of those wrinkles!

Myrrh

Frankincense

Rose

Carrot seed

Lavender

Geranium

Sandalwood

Minimize the appearance of pores and say goodbye to freckles

Lemon

Tea tree

Lemongrass

Carrot seed

Geranium

Frankincense

For the Hair

Many commercials proudly proclaim that your hair is as unique as you, but you don't find this to be a good thing when you can't find any product that does what you need it to do.

Here are the oils you want to turn to based on what you need for your hair. Blend a few drops in with your shampoo and wash as you normally would.

The results are real, and you are going to love them.

The best oily hair treatment

Lavender

Cedar wood

Peppermint

Frankincense

Sage

Basil

Clary sage

Juniper

Hair growth oils

Thyme

Lavender

Rosemary

Moisture for the dry hair

Clary sage

Lemon

Thyme

Tea tree

Cedar wood

Weight Loss and Weight Management

It seems that majority of people want to lose weight, but once they do, it is a struggle to keep it off. If you bring in these oils, you are going to see the weight melt away, as well as keep it off for good.

I suggest you use a diffuser for these oils, or that you highly dilute a drop or two into a tall glass of water. The results are real, entirely natural, and not even remotely dangerous.

You really can lose that weight for good, and enjoy the results, knowing they are going to last.

Essential weight loss

Lemon

Grapefruit

Cypress

Ginger

Peppermint

Cinnamon

Garlic

Perfect weight management

Grapefruit

Tangerine

Lemon

Spearmint

Ocotea

Cinnamon bark

Thieves

And, of course.... Peppermint

I'm sure you saw the overlap I mentioned in chapter 1 of all the ways you can use the top 3 oils, but I do strongly urge you to go out and get as many oils as you can find. They have dozens for sale on Amazon, or you can look into the other private suppliers that are around both online and locally.

No matter where you decide to get your essential oils, the important thing you need to remember is to check that they are pure. A pure essential oil is going to come in a dark bottle, as this is the best way to store them. The liquid itself is going to be strongly scented, and have an oily appearance just by looking at it.

If you get your oils from reputable sources, you have nothing to worry about, so just go through somewhere you trust, and make sure it says on the label that it is 100% pure before you buy.

Chapter 5 – The Tricks of the Trade: How to Use Essential Oils

You can know all kinds of things about essential oils, whether it be which ones are best for certain symptoms, what blends smell the best, or what kind of oils you want to avoid in various situations, but all of this is just head knowledge unless you know how to take them from the vial and put them into your life.

There are a number of different methods that people use when it comes to essential oils.

The most common are:

1. Diffusing

2. Applying topical

3. Taking internally

Let's take a moment now to look at each one, and you can decide which method you prefer for yourself, or what combination of methods you want to use. Some people choose one, others combine one or two, then there are those that use all three, the great thing about essential oils and knowing how to use them is that you can do what you want, when you want it.

Diffusing

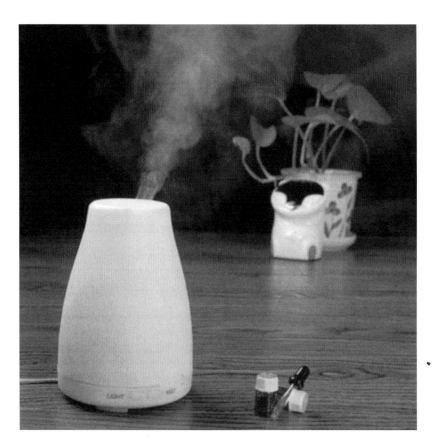

The most common method of using essential oils is diffusing. To do this, you purchase a diffuser, fill it with water (the amount of water varies with the diffuser you purchase), and add a few drops of oil.

If you know the specific symptom you want to treat, you put in the oil or blend of oils into the diffuser, plug it in, and let it fill the air with a delightful smelling mist. The aroma therapy treats the ailment, and makes your house smell incredible.

Topical use

Another prevalent method is applying the oil topically. When you do this, you still choose the oil you want based on the symptoms that are at hand. For example, you know that peppermint helps with stomach aches and lavender helps with restlessness, so if you are dealing with the stomach flu, a blend of these two oils will help a lot.

To apply topically, you are only going to use a few drops total, perhaps 2 drops of each oil.

Now, many oils are harsh applied directly to your skin, so you need to be careful with the oils you are using. The best way to prevent any skin irritation is to combine the oil with a carrier oil.

Carrier oils are mild oils that can be applied liberally to any part of your body, they are usually common oils such as coconut, sunflower, olive oil, or even vegetable oil if you are in a pinch.

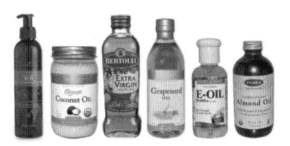

The best ratio I have found with the essential oil and the carrier oil is to combine a few drops of the essential oil with half a tablespoon of the carrier oil. Spread this on the part that is ailing (massage it into your forehead, onto your stomach, or any joint that is ailing. I find that it helps to warm the oil slightly before massaging it into your body.

Taking the Oil Internally

There is a lot of debate when it comes to ingesting essential oils. Many people advise against it because there can be harmful side effects, or you can overdose on the oils if you don't follow the dosages.

In my experience, I have never had an issue taking a couple drops of oil in my tea, but I am always careful of proper dosages. If you are going to use it in your tea, only use a couple of drops, no matter how big your cup of tea is. Only do this once a day.

Sure, there is the tendency to think that if 2 drops is good, then 4 must be better, but that is not the case. Essential oils are highly concentrated, which means the couple drops you are using in your tea is the equivalent to a lot of the fruit or other substance you are using.

Go mild, blend it into the tea you are drinking, and remember that less is more. If you feel sick, dizzy, or like something is off, discontinue ingesting the oils and simply use them topically or diffused into the air. There is evidence to support that you get the same benefits from using these oils topically or through aroma therapy as there is ingesting it.

At the end of the day, you get to decide what you want to do. It's your body, you get to decide. Don't be afraid to try out all three and decide which you want to do for yourself, and have fun with it!

My goal with this book is to give you the freedom you deserve to have with your health, and using essential oils is the best way to do that.

Conclusion

There you have it, everything you need to know to get well versed in the use of essential oils. With this book, you will know not only what kind of oils to use for certain ailments, but you will also know which blends to make and how to administer for the greatest results.

Discover your perfect method, combine that with your favorite blends, and reap the excellent benefits that are sure to follow. In no time at all you will know just what to do with any ailment that arises, no matter what time of the day it is.

I hope this book is able to show you how you can treat any ailment naturally, and you can do it your way. No strict rules, no crazy side effects to worry about, and absolutely none of that medicinal smell that you don't want on you or your children.

Natural remedies are by far the best way to go, and when you know what you are doing, you have the very key you need to make it happen. That is what this book aims to do, and that is exactly what you will be able by the time you have reached this point.

I hope you now feel the confidence I know you should have, and that you are able to treat and prevent a variety of ailments that arise in day to day living. These treatments are the best of the best. They have been around for thousands of years for a reason... they work!

Forget the stress that comes from going to the store and standing in the medication aisle for hours, trying to decide which one is best for you. Now, you can treat anything you can think of naturally, and naturally you can do it whenever you please.

FREE Bonus Reminder

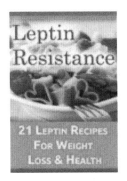

If you have not grabbed it yet, please go ahead and download your special bonus report *"Leptin Resistance. 21 Leptin Recipes For Weight Loss & Healthy Living"*.

Simply Click the Button Below

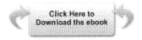

OR **Go to This Page**

http://easyweightlossway.com/free/

BONUS #2: More Free & Discounted Books

Do you want to receive more Free & Discounted Books?

We have a mailing list where we send out our new Books when they go free or with a discount on Kindle. Click on the link below to sign up for Free & Discount Book Promotions.

=> Sign Up for Free & Discount Book Promotions <=

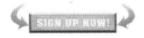

OR Go to this URL

http://zbit.ly/1WBb1Ek

Printed in Great Britain
by Amazon

67489727R00025